Wannabe Healthy

A simple Guide to Healthy Living
By: Crystal Escobar

Wannabebalanced.com

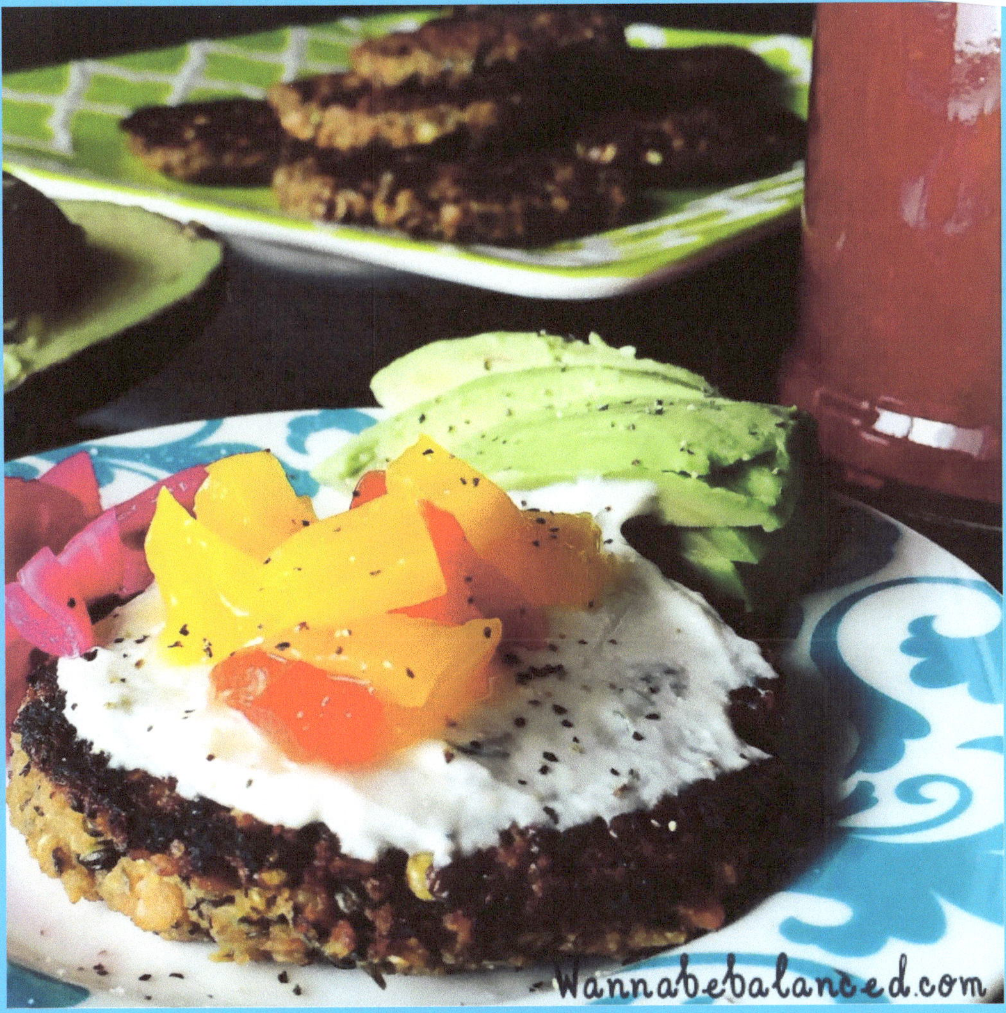

Stay Connected!

For more healthy tips and recipes be sure to follow:

Instagram: @Crystalescobar2

Periscope: @CrystalEscobar or you can find me under Wannabe Balanced Mom

Pinterest: @Crystalesco

Join our Facebook Group: @Wannabe Balanced

Text or Call: 801-792-9759

Email: crystal@escoweb.net

Visit my blog: WannabeBalanced.com

Because Everything in Life Should be Beautiful.

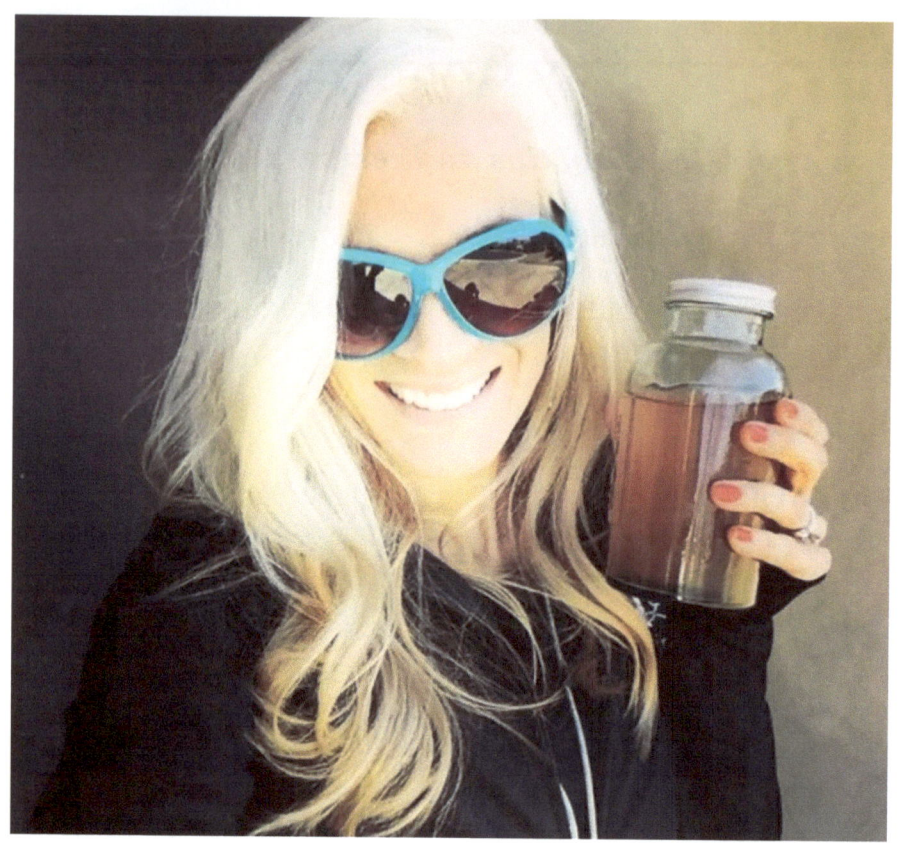

In this book I will give you my crash course guide to a healthier lifestyle. Over the last decade my diet has evolved into a nutrient dense, probiotic packed, tasty work of art. I want to show you just how easy and enjoyable it can be to eat and drink yourself to a thinner, more energetic, healthier YOU! I've learned that the 3 most important aspects of a healthier lifestyle are as follows:

1. Cultured Foods and drink (Kombucha, fermented veggies, and Kefir).

2. Sprouting and raw foods

3. Cleansing the body from the inside out.

I'll teach you how to incorporate all these things into your life with simple step by step instructions and shopping lists.

My true passion is all about helping others cultivate a healthier lifestyle by nurturing the mind, body, and spirit. I have a blog called Wannabe Balanced where I share my lifelong journey to obtaining and maintaining balance as a mom of 4 children.

I believe in God and know that our bodies are temples for our spirit, therefore we must offer the same kind of care and respect we would a sacred work of art. We need to take care of our physical bodies in order for our minds to function properly and also to reach a higher degree of spirituality. They are all connected. You cannot grow spiritually if you don't take care of your physical body. Everything must be in alignment.

My purpose in educating others about health goes way beyond the physical affects. I want to help others reach a greater level spiritually, physically, and intellectually.

For more tips, recipes, and information on events, subscribe to my blog at WannabeBalanced.com. I teach free classes on these topics and also post a lot of information on my blog and Instagram. I look forward to helping you on your journey to better health and wellness.

Crystal Escobar

Find me Periscope!
Wannabe Balanced Mom

visit my blog: WannabeBalanced.com

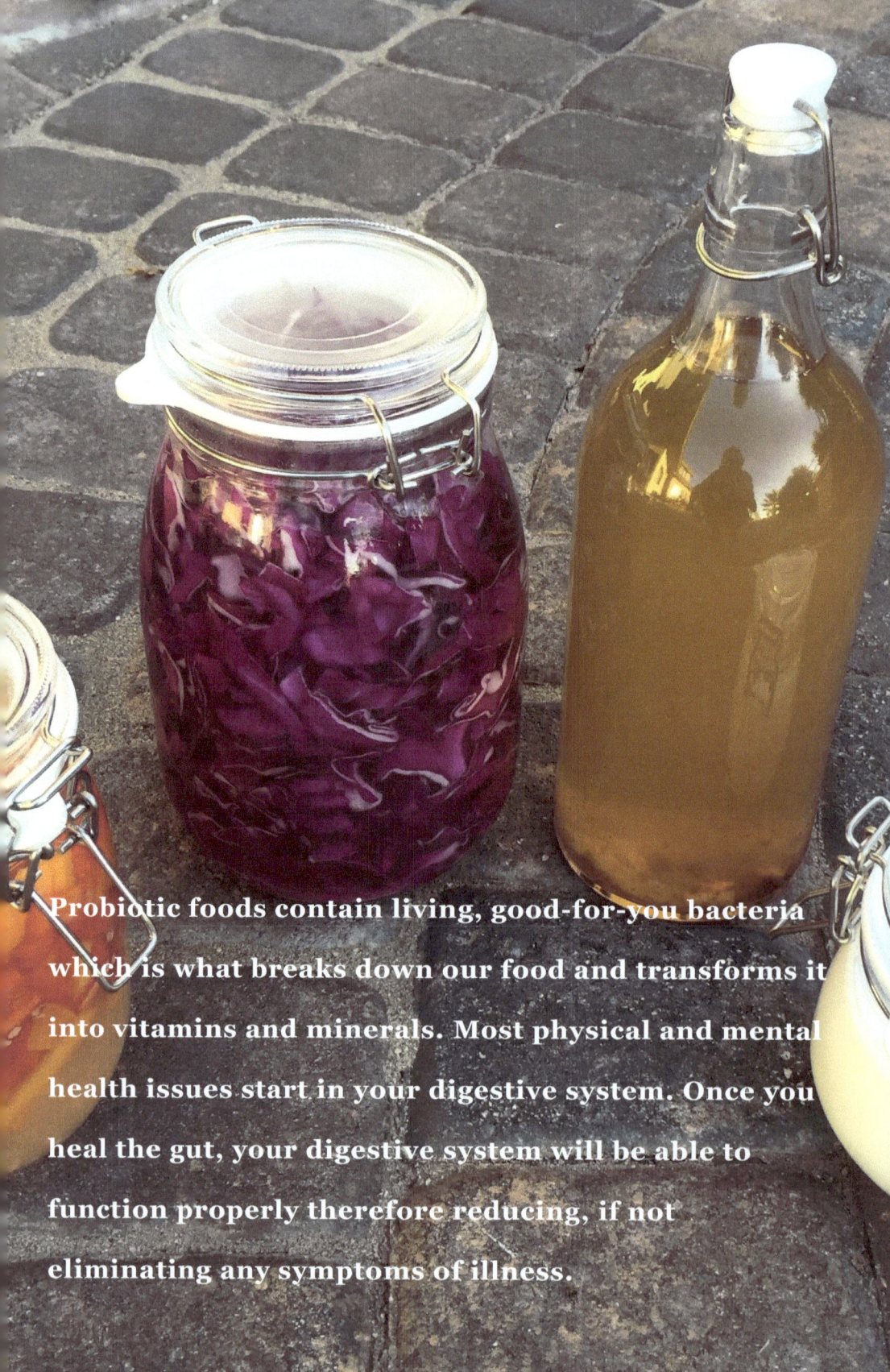

Probiotic foods contain living, good-for-you bacteria which is what breaks down our food and transforms it into vitamins and minerals. Most physical and mental health issues start in your digestive system. Once you heal the gut, your digestive system will be able to function properly therefore reducing, if not eliminating any symptoms of illness.

Noted Health Benefits:

Eliminates constipation
Helps lactose intolerance
Acts as a natural antibiotic
Supports the immune system
Enhances digestion
Helps with weight loss
Cancer prevention
Boosts energy
Combats colds and flu
Enhances mood
Stabilizes blood sugar levels

Equipment Needed:

Pint-sized glass jars

Cheesecloth, paper towel, or clean napkin

Rubber band

Small strainer (preferably plastic, but metal is ok)

Storage container with lid

Stock pot

Gallon glass jar

Tightly woven cloth, coffee filters, or paper towels, to cover the jar

Bottles: 6 swing-top bottles

Also you will need a small funnel, and fine mesh strainer

Kombucha is a beverage the ancient Chinese called the "Immortal Health Elixir?" Its been around for more than 2,000 years and has a rich anecdotal history of health benefits like improving digestion, boosting energy, reducing stress, and helping your immune system.

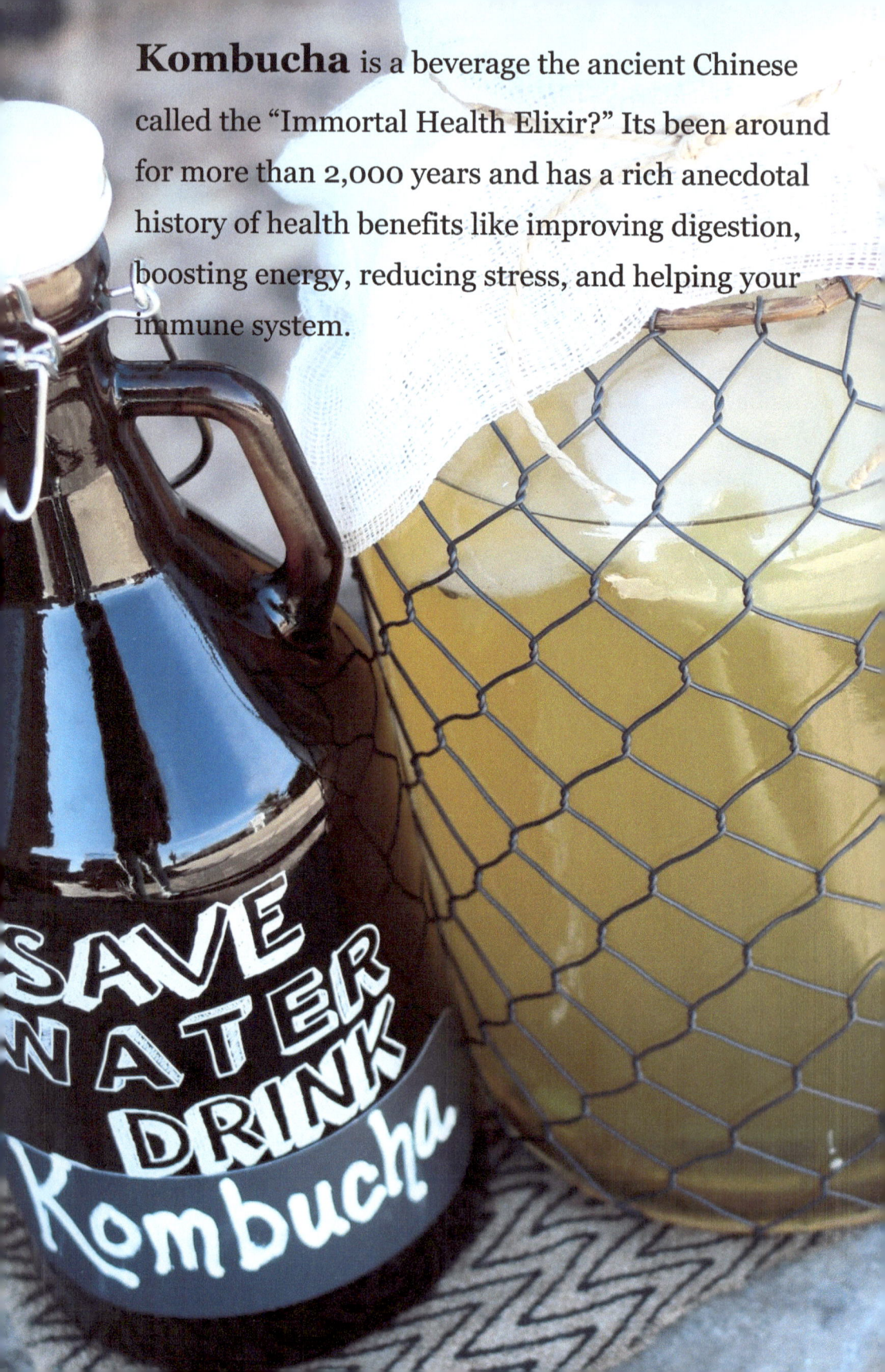

Instructions

Note: Avoid prolonged contact between the kombucha and metal both during and after brewing. This can affect the flavor of your kombucha and weaken the scoby over time.

Make the tea base: Bring the water to a boil. Remove from heat and stir in the sugar to dissolve. Drop in the tea and allow it to steep until the water has cooled. Depending on the size of your pot, this will take a few hours.

Add the starter tea: Once the tea is cool, remove the tea bags or strain out the loose tea. Stir in the starter tea/2 cups Kombucha. (The starter tea makes the liquid acidic, which prevents harmful bacteria from growing in the first few days of fermentation.)

Transfer to jars and add the scoby: Pour the mixture into a 1-gallon glass jar and place the scoby into the jar with clean hands. Cover the mouth of the jar with a few layers tightly-woven cloth, coffee filters, or paper towels secured with a rubber band.

Ferment for 7 to 10 days: Keep the jar at room temperature, out of direct sunlight, and where it won't get moved or bumped. A new layer of scoby should start forming at the top of the kombucha within a few days. It usually attaches to the old scoby. You may also see brown stringy bits floating beneath the scoby, sediment collecting at the bottom, and bubbles collecting around the scoby. This is all normal and signs of healthy fermentation. After 7 days, begin tasting the kombucha daily by pouring a little out of the jar and into a cup. When it reaches a balance of sweetness and tartness that is pleasant to you, the kombucha is ready to bottle.

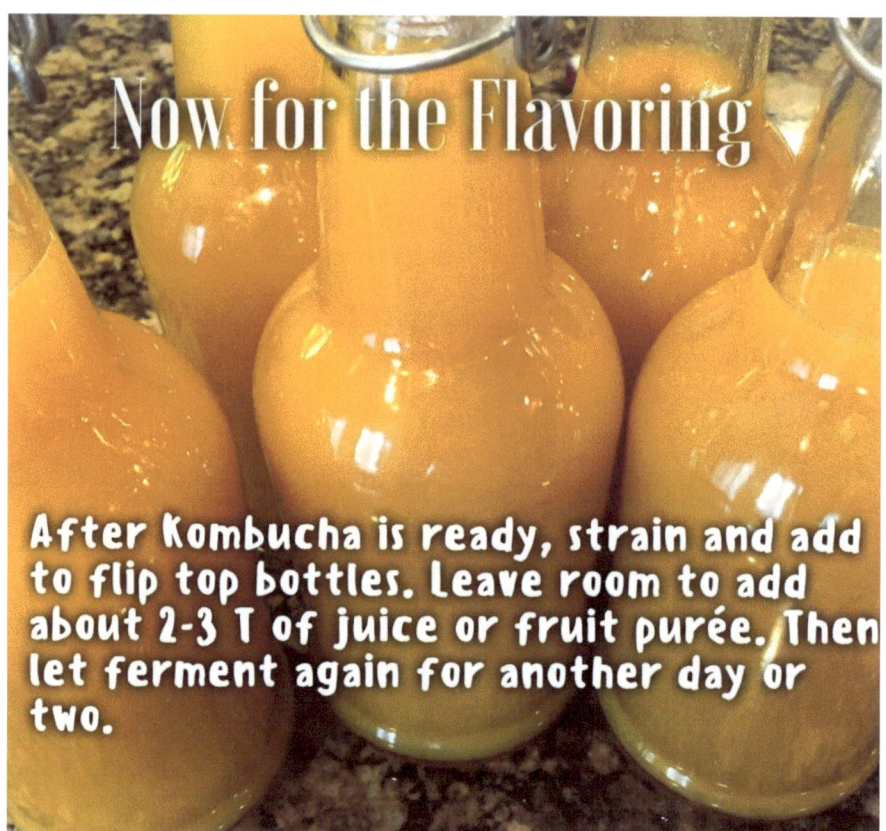

Now for the Flavoring

After Kombucha is ready, strain and add to flip top bottles. Leave room to add about 2-3 T of juice or fruit purée. Then let ferment again for another day or two.

Remove the scoby: Before proceeding, prepare and cool another pot of sweet tea for your next batch of Kombucha. With clean hands, gently lift the scoby out of the kombucha and set it on a clean plate.

Bottle the finished kombucha: Measure out your starter tea (2 cups) from this batch of kombucha and set it aside for the next batch. Pour the fermented kombucha (straining, if desired) into bottles using the small funnel, along with any juice, herbs, or fruit you may want to use as flavoring. Leave about a half inch of room in each bottle.

Carbonate and refrigerate the finished kombucha:
Store the bottled kombucha at room temperature out of
direct sunlight and allow 1 to 3 days for the kombucha to
carbonate. Refrigerate to stop fermentation and
carbonation, and then consume your kombucha within a
month.

Make a fresh batch of kombucha: Clean the jar being
used for kombucha fermentation. Combine the starter
tea from your last batch of kombucha with the fresh
batch of sugary tea, and pour it into the fermentation jar.
Place the scoby on top, cover with coffee filter, and
ferment for 7 to 10 days.

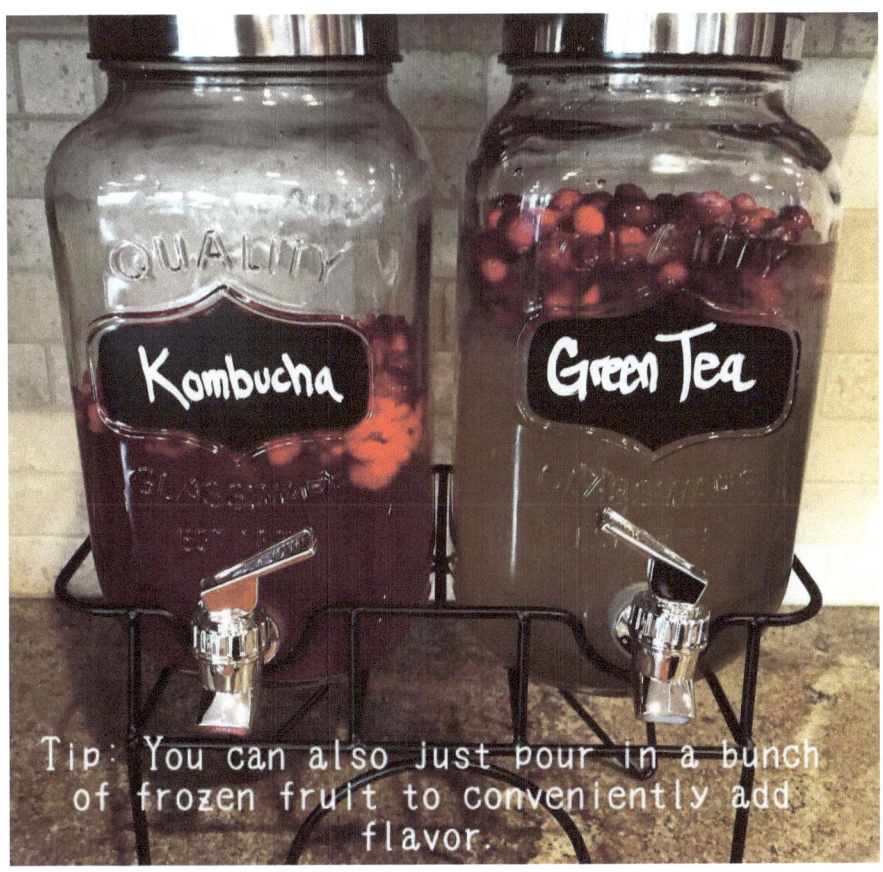

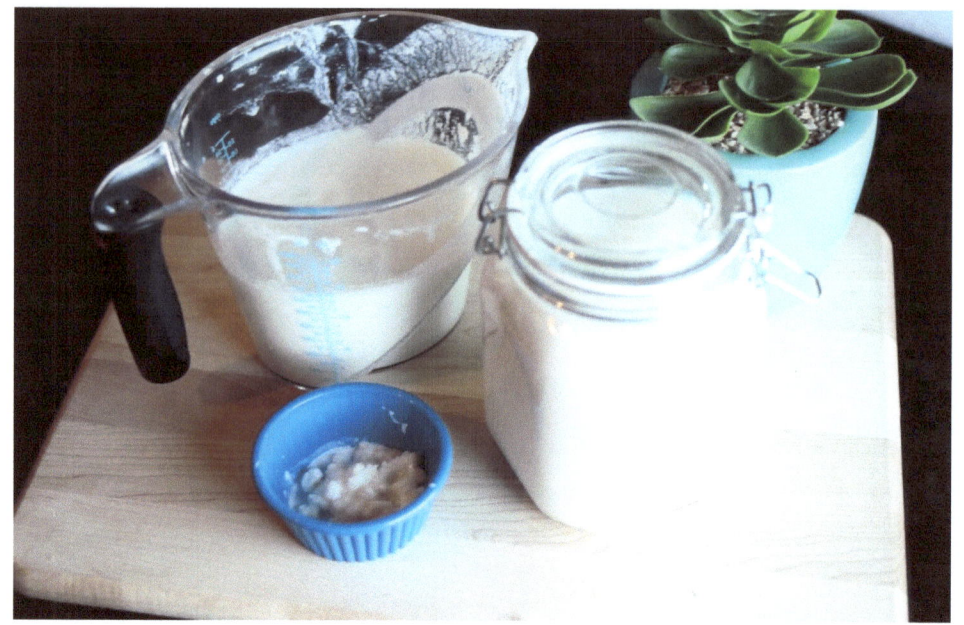

Kefir

Kefir is another way to get different stains of good bacteria into the body. It's the easiest thing to make and has endless possibilities.

All you need are Kefir grains and milk!

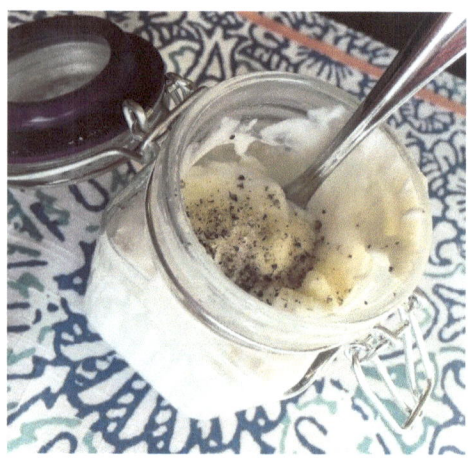

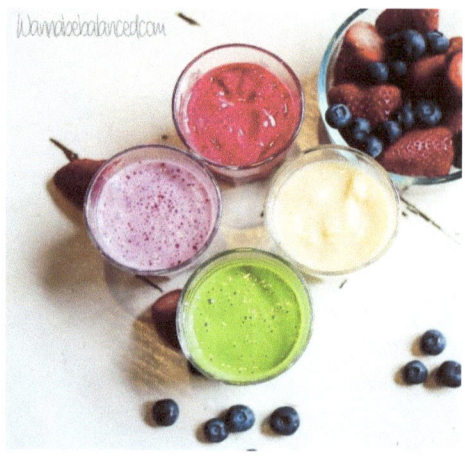

Instructions

Note: Avoid prolonged contact between the kefir and metal both during and after brewing. This can affect the flavor of your kefir and weaken the grains over time.

~Combine the milk and the grains in a jar: Pour the milk into a glass jar or cup (not metal) and stir in the kefir grains.

~Cover the jar: Cover the jar with a plastic lid, cheesecloth, or a paper towel, and use a rubber band to hold it in place.

~Ferment for 12 to 48 hours: Leave the jar out on your kitchen counter or pantry for a day or two. When the milk has thickened (looks like drinkable yogurt) and tastes tangy, it's ready. This will usually take about 24 hours at average room temperatures (between 68-72 degrees F); the milk will ferment faster at warmer temperatures and slower at cool temperatures.

~Remove the kefir grains: If you'd like to use the Kefir right away then place a small strainer over the container you'll use to store the kefir. Strain the kefir into the container, catching the grains in the strainer.

~Transfer the grains to fresh milk: To make your next batch of Kefir just stir the grains into a fresh batch of milk and allow to ferment again. This way, you can make a fresh batch of kefir every day. To take a break from making kefir, place the grains in fresh milk, cover tightly, and refrigerate.

~Drink or refrigerate the milk kefir: The prepared milk kefir can be stored in the fridge for many months but it's best to consume it within a week for optimal probiotic benefits.

Second Fermentation
Like Kombucha, Kefir can also undergo a second fermentation that improves the nutritional value as well as the taste. This process can be done with any fruit or spice. Basically all you do is add a flavor of your choice then allow to sit at room temp once again for just a few hours then place in the fridge until ready to use.

Making Kefir Cheese

Instructions:

Place a strainer in a bowl then add a coffee filter in the strainer and pour kefir into the coffee filter. Allow the whey to drain out for 12-24 hours in the refrigerator.

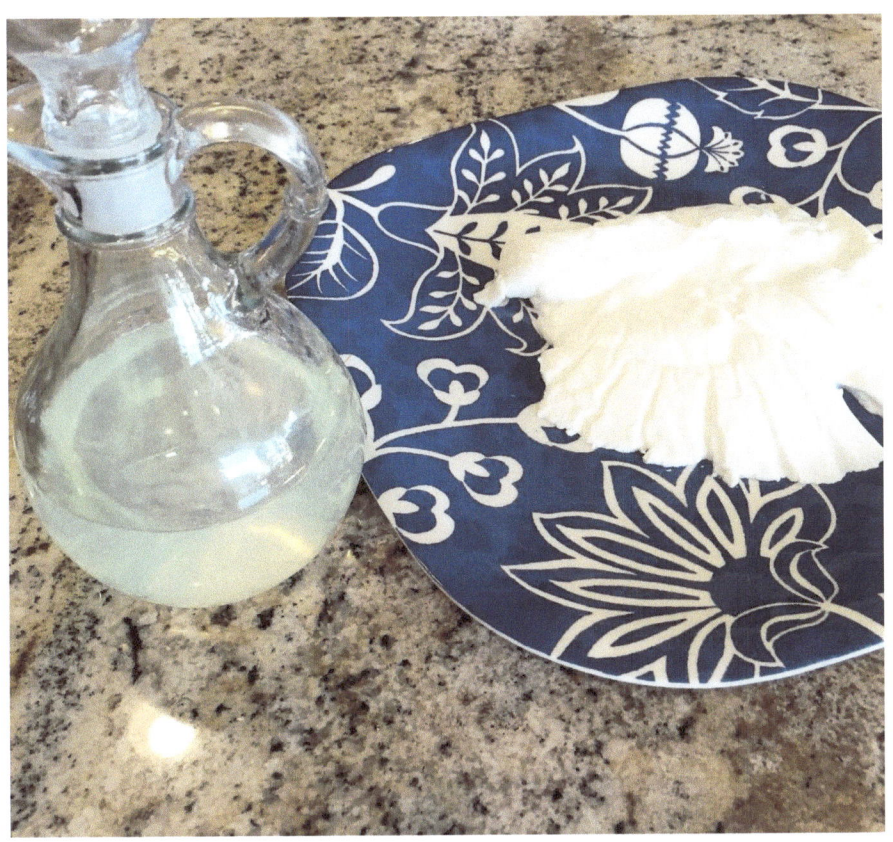

This is what the Kefir cheese will look like. Now it's the perfect consistency to create sweet or savory spreads. I like to add salt, pepper, and garlic powder to mine and spread it on crackers or toast, then top with some fermented veggies.

Do not discard the liquid whey because we are going to use it to ferment some veggies. Store it in the refrigerator until ready to use.

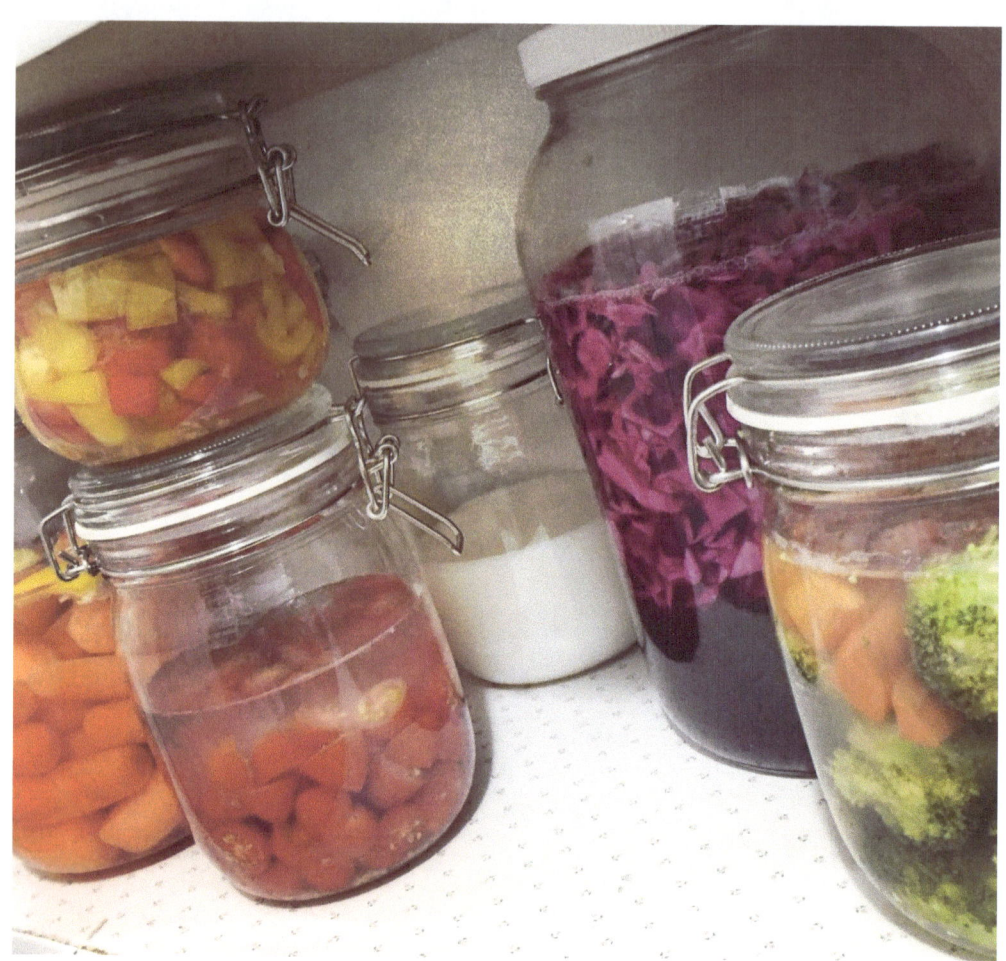

Cultured Vegetables

Fermented vegetables have been a tasty addition to my diet. Sean and I both love to top off our eggs, salads, and even my new favorite, sprouted lentil patties with a couple spoonfuls of cultured veggies.

The cool thing about cultured veggies is that they are packed full of healthy bacteria and will actually give you a nice boost of energy because of the additional enzymes and vitamin potency.

Cultured veggies have increased levels of vitamin C and good bacteria that can even remove pesticides and toxic chemicals from the vegetables.

HOW TO FERMENT VEGETABLES

1. CHOOSE YOUR FERMENTATION EQUIPMENT.
My favorite are the 1 quart flip top jars. You can find them on Amazon, or at most stores like Target or Walmart.

2. PREPARE THE VEGETABLES FOR FERMENTING.
Chop or slice up your vegetables. My two favorite fermented veggies are cabbage and bell peppers.

3. PACK VEGGIES INTO CONTAINER
You can add a little salt to the veggies for a crunchier texture. You can also add other spices and flavorings like garlic. I put a little chopped garlic in with my bell peppers and they are so yummy!

4. ADD 2 TABLESPOONS OF WHEY
Use the whey left over from making your Kefir cheese. Then fill the container with filtered water leaving at least 2 inches at the top to allow room for veggies to expand.

5. SEAL CONTAINER
Close the flip top lid and set on your counter at room temp for about 6 days.

6. CHECK VEGGIES DAILY
Make sure the vegetables are covered with the water. If they rise above at all just push them back down. If any white spots begin to form, don't worry, it's not mold. It just means that the vegetables have risen above the water. Just remove the pieces covered with the white and push the veggies under the water.

7. AFTER 6 DAYS PLACE IN THE FRIDGE
Once the veggies are done fermenting you can transfer to the refrigerator and store for up to 9 months.

Sprouting

The process of sprouting increases enzyme activity, breaks down the macro nutrients into their simplest form and multiplies the nutritional value.

WHAT TO SPROUT?

Nuts, seeds such as sunflower, radish, clover, mustard, fenugreek, broccoli, and alfalfa. Lentils, garbonzo beans, grains like spelt, wheat, kamut and rye.

HOW TO EAT THEM:

Sprouts provide extra flavor and mega nutrition to salads, casseroles, and sandwiches.

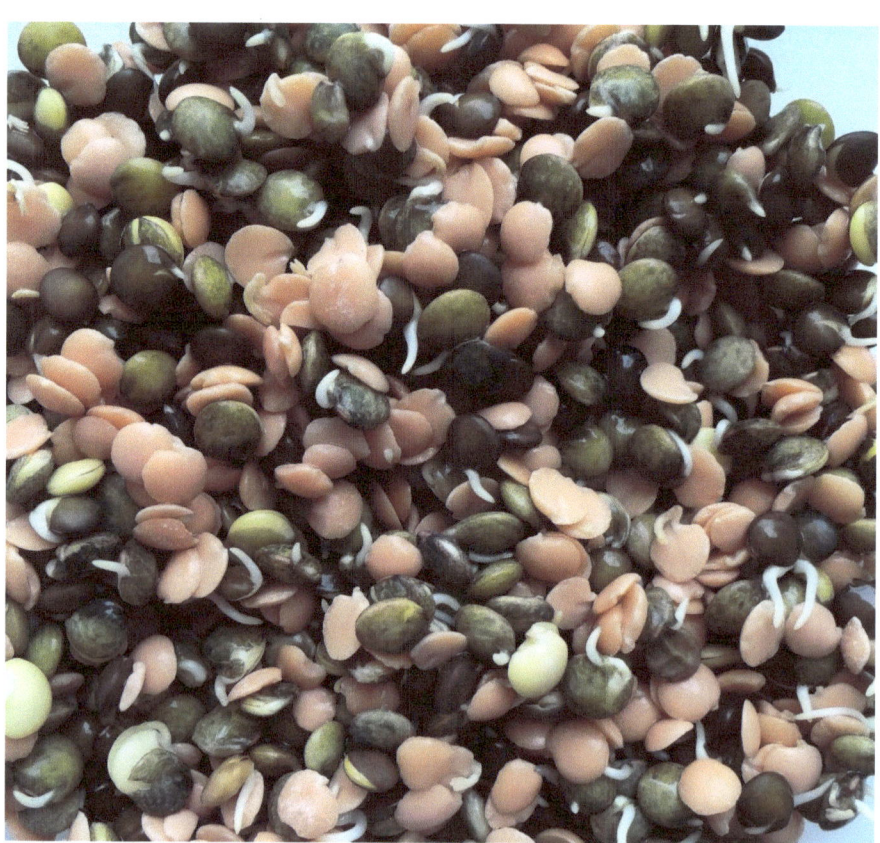

Step One:

Choose a seed, nut, or grain. Rinse well then fill the jar with filtered water and let soak over night.

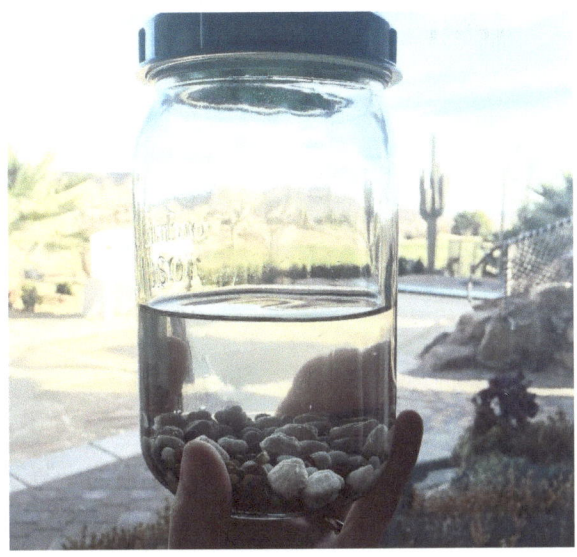

Step Two:

Drain the water and rinse 2-4 times a day. Drain well after each rinse. Position jar at a 45 degree angle. Allow sprouts to grow at room temperature for 2-7 days depending on what you're sprouting. Some things take longer to sprout.

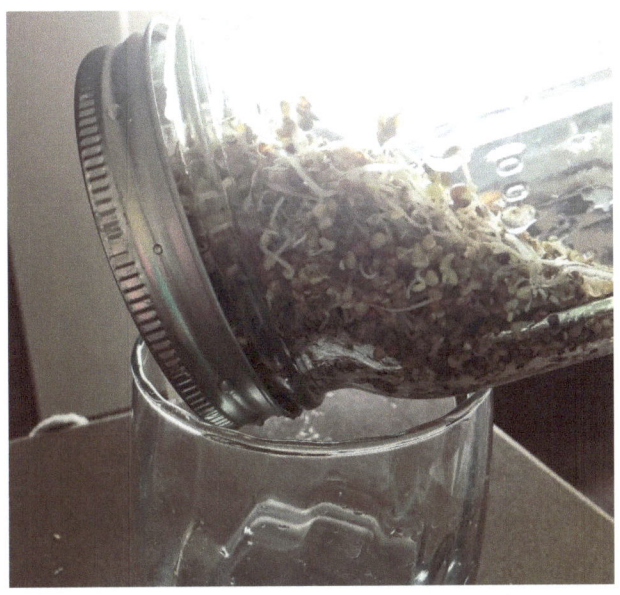

ARE YOU TOXIC?

Weight loss has become a subject too commonly spoken of over the past decade. Things are shifting though. We are becoming a more health conscious society rather than a "being skinny" obsessed people. Don't get me wrong, losing weight is still a priority for most women, especially moms. We put our bodies through so much in order to bring these little babies into the world. Then we pretty much devote all of our time and energy into raising them. Needless to say, it takes a tole on our bodies and our health. More and more we are realizing that our health can NOT be put on the back burner while we raise our children. Our health is exactly what will power us through the many hours required for caring for our family. Weight loss is great, but health is essential. That's why I'm so passionate about **Nutritional Cleansing**! Because it's not just another diet that we do for a week then fall back to our old eating habits. It's a lifestyle change that everyone can do. Just give it a week and you will see what happens. It's the perfect way to jump start better eating habits. You will first cleanse out all the toxic junk that you're body has become addicted to. Diet coke, fast food, energy drinks and sugar. Then you really are starting fresh. A clean slate. You will be amazed at how much easier it will be to do a whole 30 program, or go gluten free, or to get off that diet coke completely.

When I first did this program back 11 years ago. I had gotten to a point where I basically lost hope that I would ever be able to lose weight and keep it off. I had tried EVERYTHING! But what I didn't know back then is that we are ALL toxic. It's the sad truth but we are exposed to so many chemicals whether we like it or not. Our air is polluted, our water is polluted, our food is not only polluted but it is depleted of nutrients. These are all facts that I've learned over the years. There are multiple documentaries surrounding the subject. Sadly the majority of us are going about our lives in ignorance, just trusting the masses but not realizing that we all need to take responsibility and be proactive about our Health and get EDUCATED.

We wonder why we don't feel good, can't lose the weight, or overcome addictions. We are sick and tired of being sick and tired.

Like I said, I did my first cleanse 11 years ago before I even had kids. I was amazed with my results, but still believed that I would eventually gain the weight back. I was able to lose a total of 25 lbs and go from a size 10 to a 5. That's even smaller than I was in high school. So, as time went on and I remained consistent with the program, I never did gain any weight back. Now after having 4 kids I'm STILL back in my size 5 jeans. It's seriously a dream come true!

The weight loss is just an exciting side benefit to cleansing the body. Other things you will notice when cleansing out the junk is, getting a handle on your food cravings, increased energy, stamina, and mental clarity. We have coached thousands of people through a 30 day program and have seen all kinds of amazing results. What it all comes down to is the simple fact that it WORKS and that's why my husband and I have been able to achieve tremendous success financially. We are living our dream all because we continue to share what we KNOW with others.

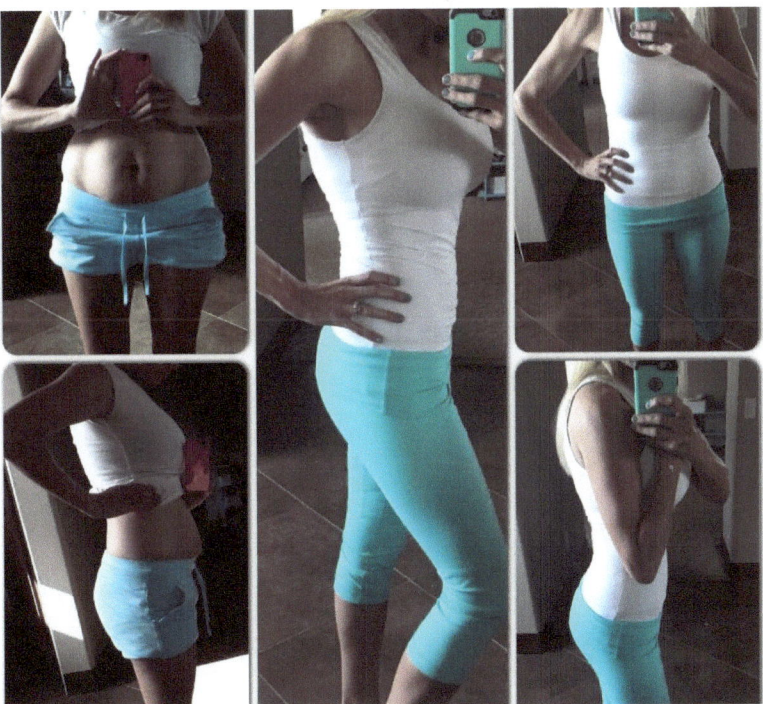

Nutritional Cleansing

Unlike a colon cleanse or laxative products, Cleanse for Life uses a synergistic blend of natural compounds to ensure the energizing nutrients flood into the body as the toxins are cleansed out.

Helps your body naturally detox and gently eliminate impurities while infusing it with vitamins, minerals, and antioxidants.

It is *not* a colon cleanse or laxative, but a nourishment product aimed to make your cleansing safe and effective. The nutrients in Cleanse for Life aid your body while it releases toxins stored in fat cells into circulation so they can be excreted.

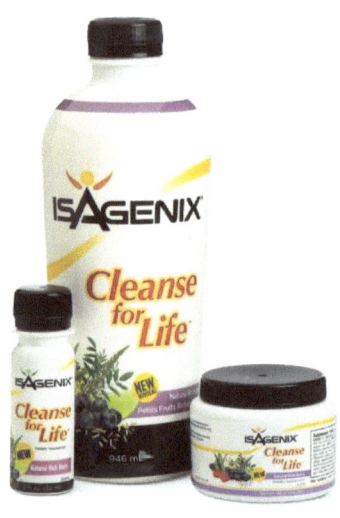

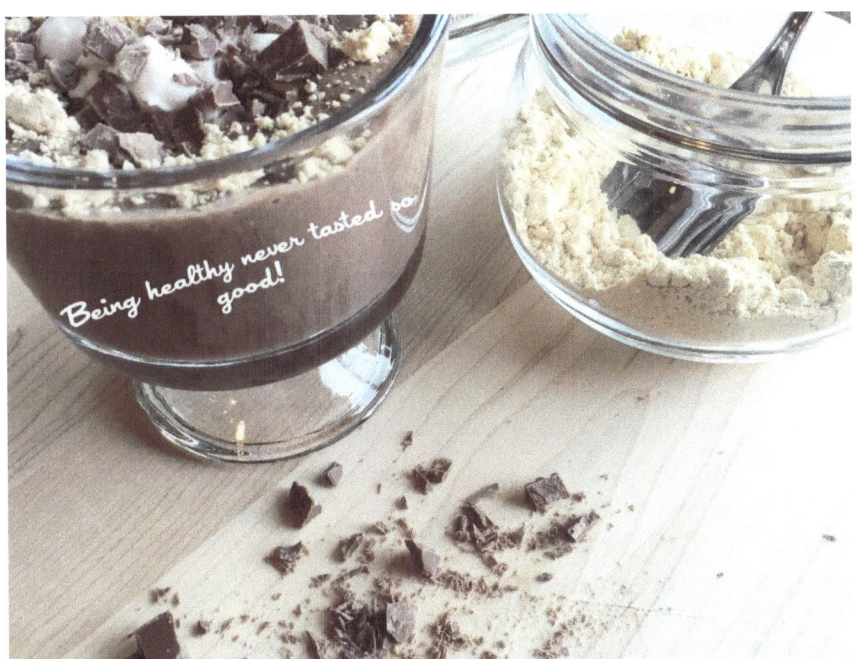

Being healthy never tasted so good!

Meal Replacement

Sometimes it's just easier to have the option of a tasty, perfectly balanced meal, ready in seconds. I cannot live without my Isalean shakes. I've had them every morning for the last 12 years. It saves me time, it's delicious, and I feel amazing after drinking it. Just one less meal to prepare which is always nice as a busy mama.

Comparing Apples to Oranges

I know there are hundreds of different meal replacement shakes out there so I wanted to give you a couple comparisons in hopes to enlighten you on what sets Isagenix apart from most other shakes. Since Shakeology is pretty popular these days I wanted to show you how they compare in quality and price.

Isagenix Whey~ Comes from grass-fed cows in New Zealand. Their whey is also undenatured, which essentially means it isn't overheated and the nutrients aren't depleted.
Shakeology Whey~ You can go to their website and read where their whey is sourced from.

Isagenix Isalean~ Comes in 2 week supples, which costs $40 a canister/$80 a month/$2.85 a shake.
Shakeology~ Only comes in a 30-day serving, which costs $130 a month/$4.33 a shake

GET CREATIVE

There are so many unique and creative ways to consume your fermented and sprouted foods. Allow me to show you some of my creations.

~Add some Kefir cheese to your guacamole.
~Make Pancakes with protein powder and Kefir.
~Try a Kombucha float by adding root beer flavor to your Kombucha and turning your Kefir into vanilla ice cream.
~Spread a little Kefir cheese on some toast and top with some fermented bell peppers.
~Make sprouted black bean patties and top with a Kefir spread, avocados, sprouted lentils and fermented bell peppers.

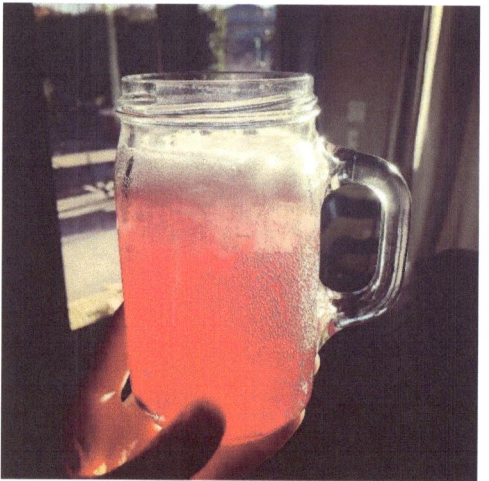

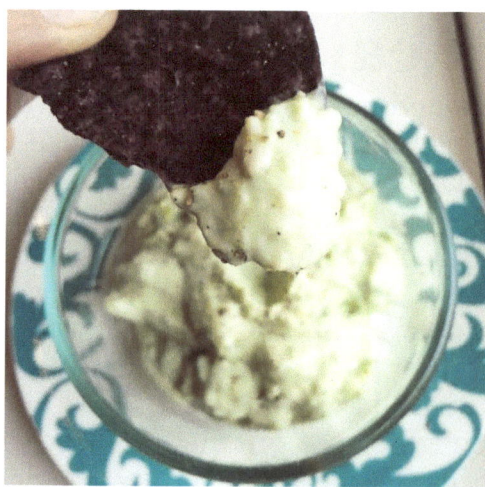

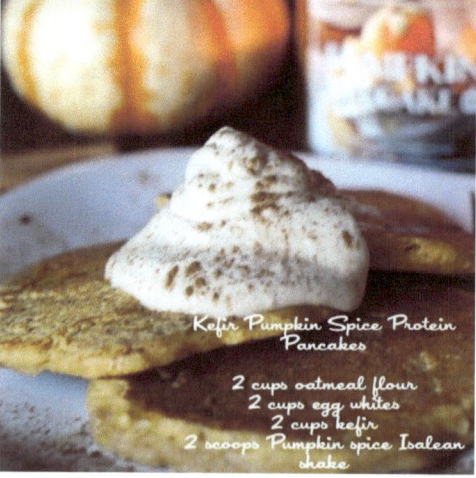

Kefir Pumpkin Spice Protein Pancakes

2 cups oatmeal flour
2 cups egg whites
2 cups kefir
2 scoops Pumpkin spice Isalean shake

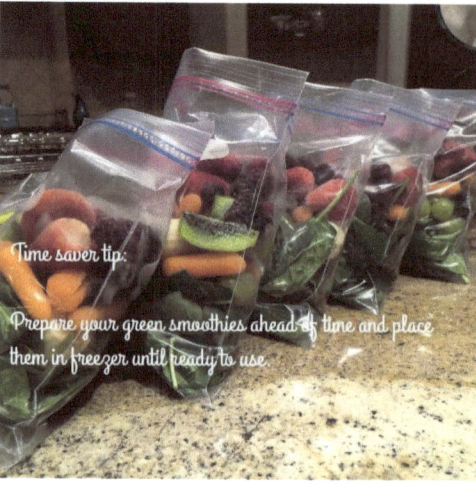

Time saver tip:

Prepare your green smoothies ahead of time and place them in freezer until ready to use.

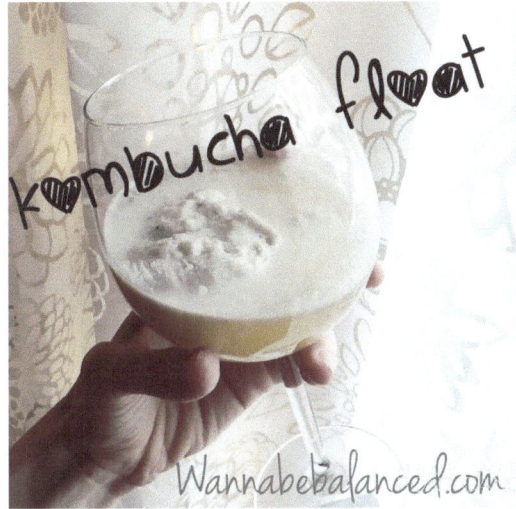

kombucha float

Wannabebalanced.com

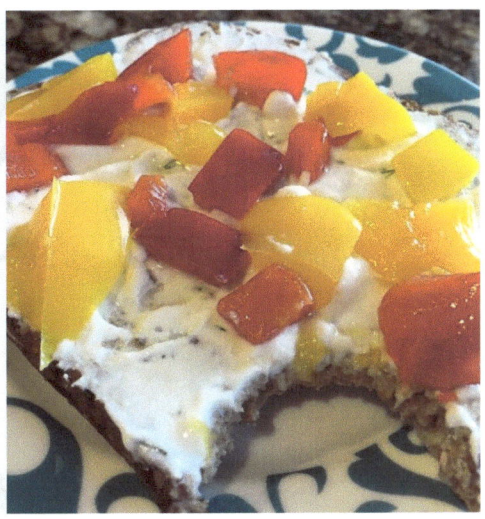

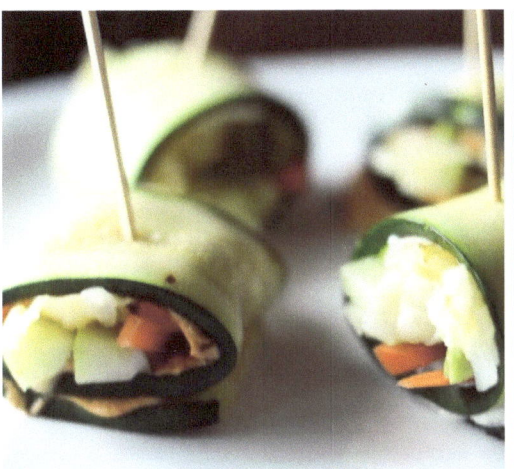

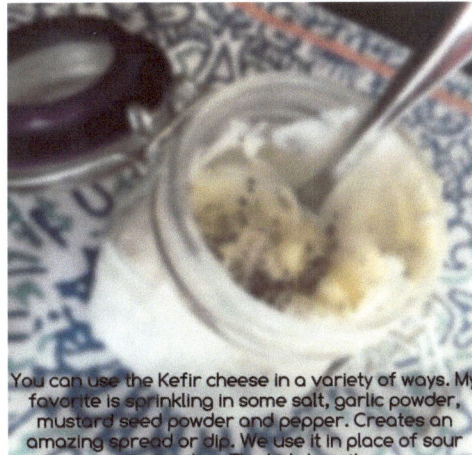

You can use the Kefir cheese in a variety of ways. My favorite is sprinkling in some salt, garlic powder, mustard seed powder and pepper. Creates an amazing spread or dip. We use it in place of sour cream too. The kids love it.

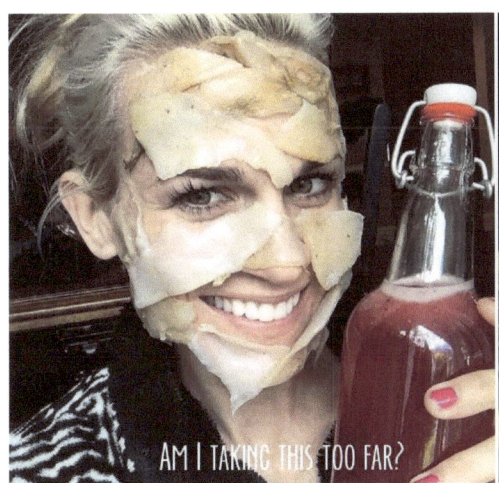

AM I TAKING THIS TOO FAR?

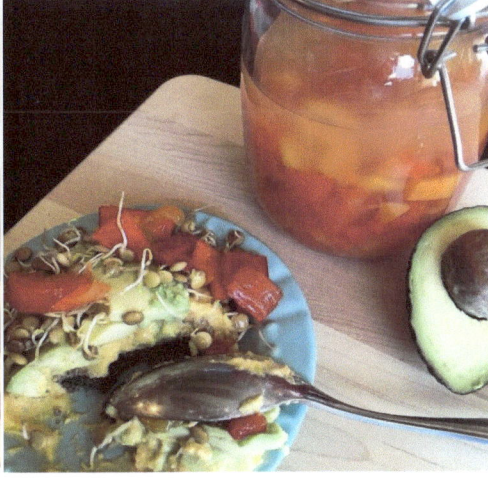